HOW TO GET STARTED ON THE NUTRISYSTEM DIET

An All-natural, Easy-to-Follow Plan to Lose Weight, Start Healthier Eating Habits and Rejuvenate Your Health

Chris Preston, RDN

ACKNOWLEDGEMENTS

I would like to express my deepest gratitude to everyone who supported me throughout the journey of creating this book. To my family and friends, your unwavering encouragement and patience have been invaluable.

A special thanks to my team, whose expertise and guidance were crucial in developing the dietary plans and recipes shared in this book. Your insights have been a cornerstone of this work.

I am also deeply grateful to my editor, Michael Jones, for your meticulous attention to detail and for helping shape this book into a comprehensive and accessible guide.

To the support groups and communities who shared their experiences and provided feedback, your contributions have enriched this book and made it more relatable for those living with fructose intolerance.

Lastly, to my readers, thank you for embarking on this journey with me. I hope this book provides you with the knowledge and tools to navigate your dietary needs and improve your quality of life.

COPYRIGHT

This book is intended to provide general information about diet and nutrition. It is not intended as a substitute for professional medical advice, diagnosis, or treatment. Always seek the advice of your physician or other qualified health provider with any questions you may have regarding a medical condition.

TABLE OF CONTENTS

ACKNOWLEDGEMENTS...2

COPYRIGHT...4

TABLE OF CONTENTS 6

INTRODUCTION TO THE NUTRISYSTEM DIET
....1

How Nutrisystem Works: Understanding the Science behind It..5

Benefits of the Nutrisystem Diet Plan...............8

Who Should and Shouldn't Consider the Nutrisystem Diet? 14

GETTING STARTED WITH NUTRISYSTEM.....17

How to Sign Up and Get Started with Nutrisystem...24

Understanding Nutrisystem Meals: What's Included and How to Customize 27

NUTRISYSTEM DIET MEAL PLANNING 36

Incorporating SmartCarbs and PowerFuels into Your Daily Meals 38

DELICIOUSLY SIMPLE RECIPES YOU MUST TRY! 41

BREAKFAST RECIPES FOR NUTRISYSTEM DIET 41

Banana oat pancakes 41

Peanut butter & date oat pots 43

Strawberry green goddess smoothie 45

Chia & oat breakfast scones with yogurt and berries 46

Cinnamon roll pancakes 49

Chocolate chip pancakes 52

Instant berry banana slush 55

Vegan tomato & mushroom pancakes 56

Rye bread with almond butter & pink grapefruit segments 58

Wholewheat flatbreads with beans & poached egg 60

Cinnamon porridge with baked bananas 63

Cinnamon twists 65

Banana & cinnamon pancakes with blueberry compote 69

Puff pastry cinnamon rolls 72

LUNCH RECIPES FOR NUTRISYSTEM DIET ..75

Healthy egg & chips 75

Braised cabbage & carrots 76

Turkey enchiladas 78

Salmon spaghetti soup with broccoli pesto.....81

Pear, blue cheese & walnut sandwich topper.85

Open rye sandwich with chicken & avocado .86

Spinach & tuna pancakes 87

Cheshire cheese, spinach & watercress salad .90

Niçoise chicken salad..92

Sticky chicken & chorizo skewers....................96

Chicken & avocado salad with blueberry balsamic dressing 100

Bean & quinoa salad with orange 102

Wild salmon with corn & pepper salsa salad105

Hummus & avocado sandwich topper 108

Easy quinoa stir-fry 109

DINNER 114

Spinach crespolini 114

Spinach & barley risotto 118

Egg wraps with black beans & rocket 120

Honey mustard grilled salmon with puy lentils
.... 123

Cod & prawn pie with saffron potatoes 125

South American-style quinoa with fried eggs
.... 129

Healthy chicken stir-fry 132

Pepper & mushroom socca pizza 135

Spicy fish stew 138

Salmon salad with sesame dressing 141

Black bean tortilla with salsa 143

Spiced chicken with rice & crisp red onions .146

One-pot vegan rice and beans 149

Hake & seafood cataplana 152

SNACKS RECIPES FOR NUTRISYSTEM DIET155

Double ginger cookies 155

Homemade vegan bagels..................................158

Flat apple & vanilla tart....................................161

Puff pastry pizzas...163

Glamorous fairy cakes 166

Easy plum jam 168

Freezer biscuits 171

Instant berry banana slush 174

Ricotta and basil pizza 175

Mozzarella, pepper & aubergine calzone 178

Spiced mackerel on toast with beetroot salsa 182

Korean fried chicken burgers 184

Vegetarian club 188

Avocado & strawberry ices 190

LIFESTYLE INTEGRATION AND LONG-TERM SUCCESS 193

Testimonials and Success Stories from Nutrisystem Users 194

PART I

INTRODUCTION TO THE

NUTRISYSTEM DIET

The Nutrisystem diet is a popular weight loss program that delivers high-protein, low-calorie, portion-controlled meals and snacks to your door every 2-4 weeks. The company claims you'll lose up to 7 pounds in your first week. After that, they claim, you'll see a 1-2 pound drop in your weight per week. Nutrisystem offers several different meal plans to choose from based on your age, gender, health conditions, and more.

The program's first week is designed to "reboot your body," and it is more restrictive than subsequent weeks. During this week, you only consume the brand's food and shakes. This weeklong program is designed for quick weight loss of fewer than 10 pounds and can be purchased without investing in a longer-term meal plan.

After the first week, Nutrisystem customers incorporate two flex meals during the week. These meals are prepared using the ingredients that you purchase. Grocery guides are provided, so customers know what foods are compliant. Restaurant meals are allowed as flex meals. Nutrisystem's NuMi app offers specific guidance for which menu items to select and which to avoid when dining out.

There is no specific meal timing, and fasting is not required for the plan. There are no particular books to buy, but the NuMi app is strongly recommended.

Core Principles and Philosophy of Nutrisystem

Founded in 1972 by Harold J. Katz, Nutrisystem is a weight loss meal delivery program. The company sells ready-made meals in calorie-controlled portions and ships them directly to customers.

Once you select a plan based on your age and sex, Nutrisystem delivers meals and snacks to your home so you don't have to think about what you're going to eat. You'll eat six times a day, and the premade meals focus on lean proteins, healthy fats, fiber, vegetables, and "smart" carbohydrates, according to the company. These carbohydrates are lower-glycemic carbs. That means they are the type of carbohydrates that break down slowly and don't spike blood sugar, according to Harvard

Health. Because everything is prepared for you, the idea is that all you need to do is eat the provided foods and you will lose weight, because you'll be cutting calories.

A Nutrisystem diet plan ranges between 1,200 to 1,500 calories per day. Men and women have different needs when it comes to losing weight, so the company offers Nutrisystem for Men and Nutrisystem for Women. The plans are similar, with both men and women instructed to eat six times a day (a mixture of meals and snacks). There are plans that provide an entire week's worth of food for you, but also plans that allow for "Flex" meals, which are those you can prepare yourself or eat out. Most plans allow for six Flex meals per week, with two Flex snacks per week for women and four for men. Nutrisystem offers a basic package of preselected foods or Uniquely Yours

Max+, which has an expanded variety of menu options plus personalized nutrition support through the app.

How Nutrisystem Works: Understanding the Science behind It

How Does Nutrisystem Work?

Nutrisystem provides most of your meals and snacks proportioned for 4 weeks. Some foods arrive frozen, while others are ready to eat. You can also add foods you buy at the grocery store to round out your meal plan.

What they send to you depends on the Nutrisystem plan you pick. Your options are:

Uniquely Yours: This is Nutrisystem's basic plan for adults of all ages.

Complete 50 for women: This plan for women over 50 claims to support women's heart health and weight loss and help reduce night sweats and hot flashes during menopause. You can opt for high-protein meals with more vegetables. You'll eat more calories early in the day, potentially leaving you less hungry throughout the day.

Complete 50 for men: Tailored for men over 50, this plan claims to help men manage their weight and fight muscle loss as they age. On this plan, you can opt for meals with higher protein. You also will get protein shakes that, along with exercise, will help you maintain muscle mass, build strength, and improve body composition, the company claims.

Diabetes: This three-tiered plan claims to aid weight loss, help manage your blood sugar, and lower your A1c, a measurement of your average blood sugar level over the previous 3 months.

Partners: This plan is for couples who want to lose weight together. Your meal selections arrive every 2 weeks rather than every 4 weeks. You can each make different food choices. You also can opt to buy larger meals designed for two people to share.

Club Advantage: In addition to meals, this plan offers round-the-clock coaching, meal plans, a flexible delivery schedule, and more.

After you select your plan, you've got another choice pick your own meals and snacks or let Nutrisystem pick your meals for you, based on their most popular offerings. They recommend this easy option, called Chef's Choice, for beginners.

Note: Women and men typically have different daily calorie needs. Nutrisystem accounts for this in their different portion sizes and slightly different prices for women and men.

Benefits of the Nutrisystem Diet Plan

Potential benefits

Additional benefits of the Nutrisystem program include its convenience and potential to improve blood sugar regulation, especially in people with type 2 diabetes.

May improve blood sugar regulation

Many Nutrisystem foods are made with low glycemic index (GI) ingredients, meaning they may affect your blood sugar less significantly than other foods.

The GI is a scale of 0–100 that ranks foods based on how quickly they increase your blood sugar levels. For example, glucose — the sugar your body uses for energy — has a GI of 100, while strawberries, which contain a little natural sugar, have a GI of 40.

Many Nutrisystem meals are made with high fiber, high protein ingredients, which is thought to help lower the GI of these foods. However, there's no information online regarding the exact GI scores of Nutrisystem foods.

Moreover, there's some debate about whether the GI is a valid system. It categorizes some less nutritious foods as low GI and some healthier choices as high GI. For example, ice cream has a lower GI score than pineapple.

How quickly a food increases your blood sugar can also be affected by the other foods you eat with it. While GI can be a valuable tool, it has some limitations.

Still, Nutrisystem D — the high protein, low GI plan for people with diabetes — has been shown to improve blood sugar regulation significantly more than a diabetes education program without accompanying meals over 3 months in one 2009 study.

Everything is done for you: There is no need to count calories, plan menus, or really worry about what you're eating day-to-day. Certain people, like busy moms and professionals, may appreciate the prepped food as one less thing to think about during the day.

It's nutritionally balanced: Meals are in-line with official recommendations for minimizing the risk of chronic illnesses, with a good balance of protein, healthy fats, carbs, and fiber. Adding healthy fresh foods, including fruits and veggies, will expand the range of nutrients you get each day.

It's flexible: Flex meals and snacks allow you to stray from packaged foods. Being able to eat out with family members may make this a bit more realistic to follow,

Transition support: Nutrisystem offers a weight-maintenance plan once you've reached your goal weight. These plans include weekend meal plans or a combination of meals and snacks. Of course, there is an additional fee for these products.

May induce weight loss: Many people have had weight loss success on the Nutrisystem diet because it is a low-calorie eating plan. The entrées and snacks associated with the diet may also help those who follow the program learn portion control. One study found that people who followed the Nutrisystem plan lost an average of 3.8% more weight over three months than a control group who received nutritional counseling and education.

Cons

The menu is limited: Prepackaged food can get tiring, even with more than 160 menu items to choose from. Not everyone is going to enjoy the taste of a mostly packaged-food diet indefinitely, and as a rule of thumb, whole, fresh foods are healthier than those that come in a paper box or plastic wrapper.

It can get expensive: Meal plans add up, especially since you're supplementing with added fruits, vegetables, lean proteins, and healthy carbs, plus six on-your-own Flex meals and additional snacks per week.

It's one-size-fits-all: Though in some instances Nutrisystem is customizable, the plan is not individualized for the specific person. The 1,200 to 1,500 calories per day is mostly recommended across the board, which may not be right for you and your needs.

It may be hard to keep up: You may lose weight in the short term, but long term, it's not clear if you will be able to maintain those results. Nutrisystem is a good quick fix for weight loss, but not a substitute for a long-term healthy diet plan. Eventually you need to educate yourself about nutrition and understand how to make your own healthy choices.

Who Should and Shouldn't Consider the Nutrisystem Diet?

Nutrisystem has a plan tailored to people who have diabetes and need to manage their blood sugar and insulin levels. It claims that you will lose 7.8% of your body weight and lower your A1c by up to 1% in 6 months. Your A1c is your average blood sugar level over the previous 3 months.

Independent research does not fully back up this claim, however. A 2017 research review in Obesity Reviews found that people with diabetes lowered their A1c by 0.3% over 6 months. The researchers do say that this is a significant reduction in A1c and call it a "promising" short-term reduction.

However, it's less than a third of what Nutrisystem claims. There's no evidence that it's helpful for people at increased risk of diabetes, such as those with prediabetes.

Who shouldn't try Nutrisystem?

You should not sign up for the Nutrisystem diet if you:

Are pregnant or breastfeeding. The diet will not adequately support your nutritional needs.

Have heart disease. The diet does not meet American Heart Association dietary guidelines.

Have celiac disease or follow a gluten-free diet for other reasons.

Have a peanut allergy. Though not all Nutrisystem foods contain peanuts, they may be made in facilities that process peanuts.

Have a soy allergy.

PART II

GETTING STARTED WITH NUTRISYSTEM

The cost of a Nutrisystem weight loss program can range from less than $300 a month to more than $400 for a monthlong supply of meals and snacks, depending on your plan. Because men tend to need more calories, the cost of the Nutrisystem for Men plan is higher, from $10.75 per day for a Basic package of preselected foods to the Uniquely Yours Max+, which starts at $13.75 a day. For women, the Basic package starts at $8.92 per day, while the most expensive option — Uniquely Yours Max+ — starts at $12.50 per day.

You need to buy your own fresh fruit and vegetables if you want to supplement your diet. Other than that, there do not appear to be any hidden costs.

Choosing the Right Nutrisystem Plan: Options and Varieties

Nutrisystem Meals

Once you've made your food selections or opted to let Nutrisystem choose for you, you sit back and wait until your order arrives in 1-10 days. You will receive breakfast, lunch, and dinner meals, as well as three snacks per day for either 5 or 7 days per week, depending on the plan you choose. Each week, you'll supplement your Nutrisystem supplies with a trip to the grocery store for foods such as:

Fresh or frozen fruit and vegetables

Protein-rich foods, such as lean meat, poultry, fish, and tofu

Bread and cereal high in fiber and low in sugar

Eggs and dairy

Nuts and nut butters

Canned and dried foods, such as beans, pasta, and rice

Cooking oil, salad dressings, and condiments

Spices, herbs, and sweeteners

The 5-day plan includes what the company calls Flex meals. These can be meals you make at home or order in a restaurant. Nutrisystem offers recipes so you can make your own meals. It also offers guidance on making healthy restaurant choices. If you choose a 7-day plan, it covers all your meals for the week; no Flex meals are required.

Nutrisystem diet week 1

If you opt for the Uniquely Yours plan, your first week will be different from those that follow. The company calls it a 'kick start' that 'primes your body for weight loss.' They claim you'll lose up to 7 pounds in these first 7 days. The company calls it '7 in 7.'

Every day, you'll eat about 1,000 calories. In addition to your regular meal, you'll get a daily shake of a protein bar that Nutrisystem says will help you control your hunger and burn fat. You will supplement what Nutrisystem provides with at least 4 servings of store-bought, non-starchy vegetables per day. Think carrots, bell peppers, and leafy greens rather than potatoes, peas, or corn. A sample menu for a day of your first week includes:

Breakfast: A Nutrisystem nut and oat bar

Mid-morning snack: A protein shake

Lunch: A protein bar

Afternoon snack: Nutrisystem popcorn

Dinner: Nutrisystem meatloaf

At least 4 servings of non-starchy vegetables, either with meals or between them

You're advised to limit exercise during this first week as your body adjusts to your lower-calorie meal plan.

Nutrisystem diet weeks 2-4

After your first week, you'll get into the next phase, which will remain the same for the rest of your time on the Nutrisystem plan. Rather than bars and shakes, you'll eat full meals that include those prepared and provided by Nutrisystem, along with supplemental food you purchase on your own. On a typical day, you'll eat the following Nutrisystem-provided foods:

1 Nutrisystem Breakfast

1 Nutrisystem Lunch

1 Nutrisystem Dinner

1-2 Nutrisystem Snacks (the number varies by plan)

Here's a sample menu for men for a day on week 2 and beyond:

Breakfast: Nutrisystem entree, along with 2 tablespoons of almonds

Mid-morning snack: Nutrisystem chocolate nut bar

Lunch: Nutrisystem entree, along with 2 ounces of chicken breast and a cup of cooked broccoli

Afternoon snack: 2/3 cup low-fat yogurt and a banana

Dinner: Nutrisystem entree, along with 2 cups of salad topped with 1/4 cup shredded cheese and 1 tablespoon reduced-fat dressing

How to Sign Up and Get Started with Nutrisystem

Once you select which Nutrisystem plan you'd like to purchase, you'll be asked to provide basic information to create an account, including your name, address, email, and phone number.

You can also input your sex, height, and current weight, which are used to provide recommendations for personalized plans on the NuMi app.

Next, you'll be prompted to build your menu by choosing which items you'd like to receive. Items are sorted into categories by meal, and you can view the nutrition facts, ingredients, reviews, and preparation required for each dish.

If you chose Chef's Choice, Nutrisystem will select an assortment of its highest rated meals and snacks for you.

Keep in mind that the number of menu selections available can vary depending on the plan that you select. For example, the Basic plan offers at least 100 items to choose from, while the Uniquely Yours Max+ provides over 160 options.

Once you've completed your purchase, your order can take up to 5 days for processing and delivery. After your first order, shipments are delivered every 4 weeks.

In addition to the provided meals, Nutrisystem also recommends adding varying amounts of certain grocery items to your weekly menu, including fruits, vegetables, whole grains, low fat dairy products, and lean proteins.

Specific recommendations are available based on your personalized plan and can be found in the NuMi app.

Additionally, Nutrisystem encourages you to aim for 150 minutes of physical activity per week as part of the weight loss program. However, exercise is not required on any plan.

Understanding Nutrisystem Meals: What's Included and How to Customize

After the initial week on the Nutrisystem diet, some foods other than those purchased from Nutrisystem are allowed. Lean proteins, vegetables, and carbohydrate options are all foods that the NutriSystem plan allows, in addition to their own packaged meals and snacks.

Pre-Packaged Meals and Snacks

Nutrisystem meals each provide around 200 calories. These include comfort-food selections such as:

Double chocolate muffins

Macaroni and cheese

Grilled chicken sandwiches

Pizza

Nutrisystem meal bars

Nutrisystem Shakes

The system's shakes ("NutriCrush" or "Turbo Shakes") contain whey protein, flavoring, sweeteners, and herbal ingredients such as monk fruit. Shakes provide around 120 calories per serving (without milk).

Lean Proteins

Nutrisystem-approved proteins are called "PowerFuels." Each serving should provide 5 grams of protein and 80 to 120 calories. Subscribers are encouraged to consume three PowerFuels per day. The list includes:

Meat

Seafood

Poultry

Plant-based protein

Low-fat dairy

Nuts

Carbohydrates

Nutrisystem provides a list of "SmartCarbs" — low glycemic carbs that provide fiber. Each serving should provide at least 1 gram of fiber and 80 to 120 calories. Women are allowed one SmartCarb daily, and men are allotted two SmartCarbs daily. The approved list includes:

Whole grains (oatmeal, whole wheat bread, whole grain pasta)

Beans and legumes (chickpeas, black beans, kidney beans)

Fruit (banana, apple, orange)

Starchy vegetables (potatoes, corn, squash, carrots)

Fruits and Vegetables

Nutrisystem customers are strongly encouraged to consume at least four servings of non-starchy vegetables daily. You can also drink low-sodium vegetable juice as an alternative. Each serving is equivalent to 1/2 cup cooked or 1 cup raw of approved veggies, which include:

Bell peppers

Broccoli

Lettuce

Green beans

Cucumbers

Asparagus

Tomatoes

Fruit is also allowed on the Nutrisystem diet and is one of the "Smart Carb" options.

Condiments, Seasonings

Foods defined as "Extras" and "Free Foods" allow you to prepare, season, and flavor your food. Approved "Free Food" seasonings should provide no more than 10 calories per serving but are unlimited on the plan. Free condiments include:

Mustard

Garlic

Ginger

Salsa

Extras

"Extras" are condiments, cooking oils, and other foods that Nutrisystem subscribers can eat. They should only provide 10 to 35 calories per serving. A maximum of three Extras per day are allowed.

Ketchup

Honey

Mayonnaise

Avocado

Sunflower oil

Beverages

The Nutrisystem diet emphasizes drinking plenty of water. There are a couple other accepted drinks as well. In addition to water, you can drink:

Black coffee

Unsweetened tea

Herbal tea

Seltzer

Alcohol

Alcohol is also allowed on Nutrisystem, but in limited quantities. You can have two servings of alcohol per week. A serving is considered:

4 ounces of dry wine

12 ounces of light beer

1.5 ounces of liquor (80–90 proof)

What You Cannot Eat

Any foods beyond what is listed as compliant and in the compliant amounts are not allowed on the Nutrisystem diet. Most foods are allowed as long as they are within compliant measurements, except non-Nutrisystem sweets.

Sweets and Desserts

Candy

Cookies

Cake

Chocolate

PART III

NUTRISYSTEM DIET MEAL PLANNING

The first week of the Nutrisystem diet is different than subsequent weeks. It calls for eating Nutrisystem pre-packaged products, including breakfast, lunch, and dinner, in addition to a Nutrisystem shake and a Nutrisystem snack product. It also calls for four or more servings of non-starchy vegetables and at least 64 ounces of water or unsweetened tea.

There are many ways to follow the Nutrisystem diet after the first week, Here is one example of how the diet might look; Nutrisystem suggests six small meals a day.

In the Nutrisystem weight loss program, you have more than 150 dishes to choose from. Meals are composed of 45–55 percent carbohydrates, 25–30 percent protein, and less than 30 percent fat, the company notes. The usual meal plan cycle is 28 days. You will eat every two to three hours, or six times a day (breakfast, lunch, dinner, and three snacks; men get an extra snack). The calories are all controlled by portion size. Here are some examples.

Breakfast Choices: include cinnamon roll, honey wheat bagel, maple brown sugar oatmeal, and a turkey, ham, and cheese omelet.

Lunch: Typical lunch options include a chicken mozzarella melt, tuna salad, red beans and rice with quinoa, and white cheddar mac and cheese.

Dinner: A dinner selection could be artichoke and spinach stuffed chicken breast, Margherita pizza, bean Bolognese, or beef stew.

Snacks and desserts: This weight loss program has plenty of snacks and desserts to choose from, including ice cream sandwiches, fudge bars, chocolate cupcakes, white cheddar popcorn, and cheese puffs.

Incorporating SmartCarbs and PowerFuels into Your Daily Meals

Lean Proteins

Nutrisystem-approved proteins are called "PowerFuels." Each serving should provide 5 grams of protein and 80 to 120 calories. Subscribers are encouraged to consume three PowerFuels per day. The list includes:

Meat

Seafood

Poultry

Plant-based protein

Low-fat dairy

Nuts

Carbohydrates

Nutrisystem provides a list of "SmartCarbs" — low glycemic carbs that provide fiber. Each serving should provide at least 1 gram of fiber and 80 to 120 calories. Women are allowed one SmartCarb daily, and men are allotted two SmartCarbs daily. The approved list includes:

Whole grains (oatmeal, whole wheat bread, whole grain pasta)

Beans and legumes (chickpeas, black beans, kidney beans)

Fruit (banana, apple, orange)

Starchy vegetables (potatoes, corn, squash, carrots)

PART IV

DELICIOUSLY SIMPLE RECIPES YOU MUST TRY!

BREAKFAST RECIPES FOR NUTRISYSTEM DIET

Banana oat pancakes

<u>Ingredients</u>

- 125ml oat milk

- 2 eggs, separated

- 1 small banana

- 100g rolled oats

- 2 tsp baking powder

- few drops of vanilla extract

- oil, we used avocado oil spray

- low-fat yogurt and fruit to top

Preparations

- STEP 1

Put the oat milk, egg yolks, banana, oats, baking powder and vanilla in a blender and process to as smooth a mixture as you can get. Whisk the eggs whites until they hold stiff peaks. Whisk 1-2 tbsp of the whites into the batter, then fold in the rest.

- STEP 2

Heat a non-stick pan over a medium heat and spray with a whisper of oil, pour about 2 tbsp of batter into the pan and cook for 1-2 mins, until the base sets and bubbles appear all over the top. Flip and cook the other side for a minute. Repeat in batches, making sure the top looks dryish before attempting the flip, or the centre will collapse.

Peanut butter & date oat pots

<u>Ingredients</u>

- 180g porridge oats

- 75g 100% crunchy peanut butter

- 40g stoned medjool dates, chopped

- 2 tsp vanilla extract

* 5 x 120g pots plain bio yogurt (or 600g from a large pot)

* ground cinnamon, for dusting

<u>Preparations</u>

* STEP 1

Tip the oats into a large bowl and pour over 600ml boiling water. Add the peanut butter, dates and vanilla and stir well. Cool, then stir through 240g of the yogurt. Dilute with a small amount of water if the consistency is a little stiff.

* STEP 2

Spoon into six glasses, then top with the remaining yogurt and dust with cinnamon. Cover each glass and keep in the fridge until ready to eat. Will keep well for up to five days.

Strawberry green goddess smoothie

<u>Ingredients</u>

• 160g ripe strawberries, hulled

• 160g baby spinach

• 1 small avocado, halved and the flesh scooped out

• 150ml pot bio yogurt

• 2 small oranges, juiced, plus ½ tsp finely grated zest

<u>Preparations</u>

* STEP 1

Put all the ingredients in a blender and whizz until completely smooth. If it's a little thick, add a drop of chilled water then blitz again. Pour into glasses and drink straight away.

Chia & oat breakfast scones with yogurt and berries

Ingredients

* 2 tsp cold pressed rapeseed oil, plus a little for the ramekins

* 50ml milk

* 1 tbsp lemon juice

* 2 tsp vanilla extract

- 160g plain wholemeal spelt flour

- 2 tbsp chia seeds

- 25g oats

- 2 tsp baking powder

- 2 x 120g pots bio Greek yogurt

- 400g strawberries, hulled and sliced

<u>Preparations</u>

- STEP 1

Heat oven to 200C/180C fan/gas 6 and line the base of 4 x 185ml ramekins with a disc of baking parchment and oil the sides with the rapeseed oil. Measure the milk in a jug and make up to 300ml with water. Stir in the lemon juice, vanilla and the

2 tsp oil. Mix the flour, seeds and oats then blitz in a food processor to make the mix as fine as you can. Stir in the baking powder.

• STEP 2

Pour in the liquid, then stir in with the blade of a knife until you have a very wet batter like dough. Spoon evenly into the ramekins then bake on a baking sheet for 20 mins until risen – they don't have to be golden but should feel firm. Cool for a few mins then run a knife round the inside of the ramekins to loosen the scones then carefully ease out.

• STEP 3

The scones can be eaten immediately or cooled and stored for later.

Cinnamon roll pancakes

<u>**Ingredients**</u>

- 145g self-raising flour

- 1 tsp baking powder

- 1 tbsp golden caster sugar

- 1 tsp cinnamon

- 2 eggs

- 40g butter, melted

- 140ml milk

- 3 tbsp light brown soft sugar

- 1 tbsp maple syrup, plus extra to serve (optional)

- 1 tbsp vegetable oil

- 6 tbsp toffee or caramel yogurt, to serve (optional)

<u>Preparations</u>

- STEP 1

Weigh the flour in a large jug or bowl. Add the baking powder, caster sugar, ½ tsp cinnamon and a generous pinch of salt. Whisk to combine. Crack in the eggs, add ½ the butter and all the milk, then whisk to a smooth batter. Will keep in the fridge overnight.

- STEP 2

Stir the rest of the cinnamon, the light brown sugar and the maple syrup into the remaining melted butter. Add 3 tbsp of the pancake mixture and mix. Transfer to a squeezy bottle fitted with a small nozzle or a piping bag.

• STEP 3

When you're ready to cook, pour a little oil in your largest frying pan, and wipe out any excess with some kitchen paper. Keeping the pan over a low-medium heat, spoon 2-3 tbsp mounds into the pan for each pancake, leaving space for them to expand as they cook. You should get three or four in at a time. Use the cinnamon mixture in your bottle or piping bag to pipe swirls on top of each pancake. When the pancakes start to set around the edges and you see bubbles appear on top, carefully flip and cook for another 2-3 mins until golden and cooked through. Keep warm in a low oven while you continue cooking the rest of the batter.

- STEP 4

Serve the pancakes with yogurt and extra maple syrup, if you like.

Chocolate chip pancakes

<u>Ingredients</u>

- 300g self-raising flour

- 1 tsp baking powder

- 3 tbsp caster sugar

- 2 medium eggs

- 300ml whole milk

- 150g milk chocolate chips

• butter, for frying

• whipped cream or ice cream, to serve (optional)

Preparations

• STEP 1

Sieve the flour, baking powder and ¼ tsp salt into a large mixing bowl. Add the caster sugar and stir until well combined.

• STEP 2

Whisk the eggs and milk together in a jug. Make a well in the centre of the dry ingredients and pour in the wet ingredients. Use a whisk to combine everything and create a smooth batter. Fold through most of the chocolate chips.

- STEP 3

Heat a small knob of butter in a large non-stick frying pan over a medium heat, swirling it round to coat the pan. Add 2-3 tbsp of the batter to the pan and cook for 1-2 mins, or until bubbles begin to rise to the surface. Flip the pancake over and cook for 2 mins on the other side for the same amount of time, or until golden brown and puffed up. Repeat with the remaining batter, keeping the pancakes warm in a low oven.

- STEP 4

Stack the pancakes on plates and top with any leftover chocolate chips and a dollop of whipped cream or ice cream, if you like.

Instant berry banana slush

Ingredients

- 2 ripe bananas

- 200g frozen berry mix (blackberries, raspberries and currants)

Preparations

- STEP 1

Slice the bananas into a bowl and add the frozen berry mix. Blitz with a stick blender to make a slushy ice and serve straight away in two glasses with spoons.

Vegan tomato & mushroom pancakes

<u>Ingredients</u>

- 140g white self-raising flour

- 1 tsp soya flour

- 400ml soya milk

- vegetable oil, for frying

For the topping

- 2 tbsp vegetable oil

- 250g button mushrooms

- 250g cherry tomatoes, halved

- 2 tbsp soya cream or soya milk

- large handful pine nuts

- snipped chives, to serve

Preparations

- STEP 1

Sift the flours and a pinch of salt into a blender. Add the soya milk and blend to make a smooth batter.

- STEP 2

Heat a little oil in a medium non-stick frying pan until very hot. Pour about 3 tbsp of the batter into the pan and cook over a medium heat until bubbles appear on the surface of the pancake. Flip the pancake over with a palette knife and cook the other side until golden brown. Repeat with the remaining batter, keeping the cooked pancakes warm as you go. You will make about 8.

• STEP 3

For the topping, heat the oil in a frying pan. Cook the mushrooms until tender, add the tomatoes and cook for a couple of mins. Pour in the soya cream or milk and pine nuts, then gently cook until combined. Divide the pancakes between 2 plates, then spoon over the tomatoes and mushrooms. Scatter with chives.

Rye bread with almond butter & pink grapefruit segments

Ingredients

• 4 tbsp almond butter (make your own with the 'goes well with' recipe, right)

• 1 grapefruit (you will need about 100g flesh)

• 2 slices rye bread, toasted (optional)

Preparations

• STEP 1

Toast your rye bread, if you like. Segment the grapefruit and spoon the fruit, along with any juice, into a small bowl.

• STEP 2

Spread the almond butter onto the rye bread, and top with the grapefruit, drizzling any juice over the top.

Wholewheat flatbreads with beans & poached egg

<u>Ingredients</u>

- 2 eggs

For the beans

- 500g carton passata

- 2 small onions, quartered

- 1 medjool date, stoned

- 3 tsp smoked paprika

- 1 tsp balsamic vinegar

- 400g can haricot beans, drained

For the flatbreads

• 100g wholewheat flour

• ½ tsp baking powder

• 100g natural yogurt

Preparations

• STEP 1

Tip the passata into a food processor with the onions, date and paprika, and blitz until completely smooth. Heat in a medium pan, cover and simmer for 10 mins, stirring frequently, to make a thick pulpy sauce. Taste to make sure the onion is fully cooked. If not, add a splash of water and cook a little longer. Stir in the vinegar and beans, then remove from the heat.

- STEP 2

To make the flatbreads, tip the flour and baking powder into a bowl, then stir in the yogurt to make a soft dough. Tip out onto a lightly floured surface and lightly knead, fully incorporating any flour left in the bowl. Halve the mixture and flatten each piece to a rough oval, using your hands or a rolling pin, to a thickness of two £1 coins. Cut slashes through the centre of the ovals a couple of times with a sharp knife, being careful not to cut through an edge.

- STEP 3

Heat a large, non-stick pan, add a flatbread and cook for 1 min each side until firm and slightly puffed, then repeat with the other. Meanwhile, heat a large pan of water and poach the eggs to your liking.

• STEP 4

Warm the beans and serve on top of each flatbread with a poached egg and some black pepper.

Cinnamon porridge with baked bananas

<u>Ingredients</u>

• 80g porridge oats

• 150ml semi-skimmed milk

• ½ tsp ground cinnamon

• 1 large ripe banana (120g), halved lengthways and cut in half

• ½ orange, zested and juiced

* 200g plain bio yogurt

* 2 tsp toasted three-seed mix

Preparations

* STEP 1

Put the oats, milk, 450ml water and cinnamon in a pan. Bring to the boil, then turn the heat to low, stirring often, for 5 mins until thickened.

* STEP 2

Meanwhile, put the bananas in a dish with the orange zest and juice. Cover and microwave on high for 1½-2 mins until softened. Tip the porridge into bowls and top with the yogurt, banana and seeds.

Cinnamon twists

<u>Ingredients</u>

- 275g whole milk

- 40g unsalted butter, cubed

- 500g strong white flour, plus extra for dusting

- 7g dried active yeast

- 50g caster sugar

- 1 small egg, plus 1 egg, beaten, for glazing

For the filling

- 75g butter, melted

- 150g caster sugar

• 3 tsp ground cinnamon

For the coating

• 50g caster sugar

• 1 tsp ground cinnamon

Preparations

• STEP 1

Heat the milk and butter in a small pan until the butter has melted. Allow to cool slightly – the milk should be warm, not hot. Put the flour in a large mixing bowl with a pinch of salt to one side of the bowl. Add the yeast into the flour on the other side of the bowl, so it's not touching the salt. Pour in the sugar, then mix it all together.

- STEP 2

Gradually pour the warm milk into the dry ingredients, mixing with your hands until you have a relatively sticky dough. You may not need all of the milk. Add in the egg and continue to work until combined.

- STEP 3

Lightly dust a surface with flour and tip out the dough. It will be quite wet – the more you knead it, the easier it will become. Knead for around 10 mins until you have a smooth dough. Put in a lightly floured bowl to prove for 1 hr or until doubled in size.

- STEP 4

To make the filling, mix the melted butter, sugar and cinnamon together until you get a smooth paste. Set aside.

• STEP 5

Roll out the dough on a lightly floured surface to around a 30 x 40cm rectangle. Spread over the filling using a palette knife until the dough is completely covered.

• STEP 6

Fold in half widthways and cut into 16-18 strips down the shortest side. Twist both ends of each strip in opposite directions until a spiral shape forms. Holding one end in your hand, wrap the rest of the dough around it and over, pressing the ends into the bottom of the bun so it doesn't unravel during cooking.

* STEP 7

Lay on two lined baking trays spaced 5cm apart. Leave to prove for 30-45 mins until risen slightly. Heat the oven to 190C/170C fan/gas 5. Brush the tops of the buns with a little egg and bake for 18-20 mins until golden. Don't worry if a little cinnamon butter comes out.

* STEP 8

For the coating, mix together the sugar and cinnamon. Whilst still warm, toss the buns in the sugar and eat straight away.

Banana & cinnamon pancakes with blueberry compote

<u>Ingredients</u>

* 65g wholemeal flour

* 1 tsp ground cinnamon, plus extra for sprinkling

* 2 egg, plus 2 egg whites

* 100ml whole milk

* 1 small banana, mashed

* ½ tbsp rapeseed oil

* 320g blueberries

* few mint leaves, to serve

Preparations

* STEP 1

Tip the flour and cinnamon into a bowl, then break in the whole eggs, pour in the milk and whisk together until smooth. Stir in the banana. In a separate bowl, whisk the egg whites until light and fluffy, but not completely stiff, then fold into the pancake mix until evenly incorporated.

• STEP 2

Heat a small amount of oil in a large non-stick frying pan, then add a quarter of the pancake mix, swirl to cover the base of the pan and cook until set and golden. Carefully turn the pancake over with a palette knife and cook the other side. Transfer to a plate, then carry on with the rest of the batter until you have four.

• STEP 3

To make the compote, tip the berries in a non-stick pan and heat gently until the berries just burst but hold their shape. Serve two warm pancakes with half the berries, then scatter with the mint leaves and sprinkle with a little cinnamon. Chill the remaining pancakes and compote and serve the next day. You can reheat them in the microwave or in a pan.

Puff pastry cinnamon rolls

Ingredients

- 1½ tbsp ground cinnamon

- 3 tbsp caster sugar

- 320g ready-rolled puff pastry

- plain flour, for dusting

- 1 medium egg, beaten

- 50g icing sugar

Preparations

- STEP 1

Heat the oven to 200C/180C fan/gas 6 and line large baking tray with baking parchment. Stir the cinnamon and sugar together in a small bowl. Unravel the puff pastry on a lightly floured work surface, then sprinkle the cinnamon sugar mixture all over the top. Gently level the cinnamon sugar mixture with the back of a spoon so it covers the pastry almost completely, leaving a 1cm border on one of the short sides. Brush a little of the beaten egg over the exposed pastry border.

- STEP 2

Roll the pastry up in a tight log from the short side without the border. Gently press along the egg-washed border to seal, then slice into 12 equal rounds. Arrange the cinnamon rolls on the prepared baking tray, placing them up against each other so they're just touching. Brush the remaining beaten egg all over the tops and sides of the pastry, then bake for 15-18 mins until golden and risen. Leave to cool on the tray for 10-15 mins.

• STEP 3

Combine the icing sugar with 1½ tsp water in a small bowl until you have a thick icing that easily runs off the spoon. Drizzle this over the warm rolls, then immediately serve.

LUNCH RECIPES FOR NUTRISYSTEM DIET

Healthy egg & chips

Ingredients

- 500g potatoes, diced

- 2 shallots, sliced

- 1 tbsp olive oil

- 2 tsp dried crushed oregano or 1 tsp fresh leaves

- 200g small mushroom

- 4 eggs

Preparations

- STEP 1

Heat oven to 200C/fan 180C/gas 6. Tip the potatoes and shallots into a large, non-stick roasting tin, drizzle with the oil, sprinkle over the oregano, then mix everything together well. Bake for 40-45 mins (or until starting to go brown), add the mushrooms, then cook for a further 10 mins until the potatoes are browned and tender.

- STEP 2

Make four gaps in the vegetables and crack an egg into each space. Return to the oven for 3-4 mins or until the eggs are cooked to your liking.

Braised cabbage & carrots

<u>Ingredients</u>

• small knob butter

• 2 carrots, cut into batons

• 1 Savoy cabbage, cut into 8 wedges attached at the core

• 100ml chicken stock

Preparations

• STEP 1

Heat the butter in a pan, then add the carrots and sizzle for 1 min until glossy and coated. Nestle the cabbage wedges snugly in the pan and pour over the stock. Cover with a lid and simmer for 30 mins until the cabbage has wilted and the carrots are tender.

Turkey enchiladas

<u>Ingredients</u>

- 1 tbsp sunflower oil

- 500g turkey mince (2% fat)

- 1 medium onion, finely chopped

- 1 yellow pepper, deseeded and thinly sliced

- 400g can chopped tomatoes

- 400g can red kidney beans in chilli sauce

- 1 tbsp fresh lime or lemon juice

- 2 heaped tbsp roughly chopped coriander, plus extra to garnish

* 6 regular or 8 mini flour tortillas

* 50g reduced-fat mature cheddar, coarsely grated

* large mixed salad, to serve

<u>Preparations</u>

* STEP 1

Heat oven to 200C/180C fan/gas 6. Heat most of the oil in a large non-stick frying pan. Fry the turkey, onion and pepper for 5 mins, stirring regularly and breaking up the mince with a wooden spoon. Add the chopped tomatoes and kidney beans.

* STEP 2

Bring to a gentle simmer and cook for 10 mins, stirring regularly. Remove from the heat and stir in the lime juice and coriander. Season well.

• STEP 3

Lightly grease a shallow ovenproof dish with the remaining oil. Put 1 tortilla in the dish and top with a couple of generous spoonfuls of the turkey mixture. Roll up and push to one side of the dish. Repeat with the other tortillas, then spoon any remaining turkey mixture down the sides of the dish.

• STEP 4

Sprinkle the tortillas with the cheese and bake for 15 mins. Scatter coriander over the enchiladas and serve with a salad.

Salmon spaghetti soup with broccoli pesto

Ingredients

- 1 tbsp olive or rapeseed oil

- 320g carrots, finely diced

- 165g celery, finely diced

- 2 onions, finely chopped (320g)

- 2 large garlic cloves, finely grated

- 1/2 tsp dried oregano

- 2 tsp vegetable bouillon powder

- 400g can chopped tomatoes

- 2 tbsp tomato purée

• 100g wholemeal spaghetti

• 400g can cannellini beans

• 460g wild salmon fillets, skinned and cut into chunks

For the broccoli pesto

• 185g broccoli, cut into florets, stalks chopped

• 15g fresh basil, plus a few leaves

• 1 tbsp lemon juice, plus finely grated zest of 1/2 (optional)

• 1 tbsp olive or rapeseed oil

Preparations

• STEP 1

Heat the oil in a large deep-sided frying pan and fry the carrots, celery and onions over a medium heat for 8-10 mins until softened. Tip in the garlic, oregano and bouillon, then pour in 1 litre boiling water and the chopped tomatoes. Stir in the tomato purée, then cover and simmer for 10 mins.

• STEP 2

Break in the spaghetti (snap it into about three lengths), tip in the beans along with the water from the can, and simmer for 10 mins more.

• STEP 3

Stir in the chunks of salmon, then reduce the heat to low, cover and simmer for 5 mins.

• STEP 4

Meanwhile, for the pesto, cook the broccoli in boiling water for 5 mins, then cool quickly in a bowl of cold water. Drain well, then return to the bowl and use a hand blender to blitz it with the basil, lemon juice and olive oil to make a thick pesto.

• STEP 5

Ladle half the spaghetti mixture into two bowls and top with half the pesto. Scatter with some of the lemon zest, if you like, and a few basil leaves before serving. Cover and chill the remaining portions to serve another day. Will keep chilled for up to three days, or frozen for up to a month. Defrost thoroughly before reheating until piping hot.

Pear, blue cheese & walnut sandwich topper

Ingredients

- 25g blue cheese, or vegetarian alternative

- 1 small pear, sliced

- a big handful watercress

- 2 walnut halves, chopped

- slice wholegrain seeded bread or rye, or wholegrain pitta, to serve

Preparations

- STEP 1

Top bread or fill pitta with cheese, pear, watercress and walnuts.

Open rye sandwich with chicken & avocado

Ingredients

- 2 tbsp guacamole

- 2 slices rye bread

- 8 slices of tomato

- 2 Cajun grilled chicken breasts

- squeeze of lime

Preparations

- STEP 1

Divide guacamole between rye bread, spreading it evenly. Arrange 4 slices of tomato on each sandwich, and top with a sliced Cajun grilled chicken breast. Finish with lime juice and some ground black pepper.

Spinach & tuna pancakes

<u>Ingredients</u>

• 2 tsp rapeseed oil

• 2 garlic cloves, chopped

• 250g baby spinach

• 1 tbsp tomato purée

• 120g can tuna steak in spring water, drained

• 200g cottage cheese

• 2 large eggs

- 4 tbsp plain wholemeal flour

For the salad

- 200g can sweetcorn (no added salt or sugar), rinsed and drained

- 1 small red onion, finely chopped

- 85g cherry tomatoes, quartered

- 10 basil leaves, chopped

- 4 pitted Kalamata olives, sliced

- 2 tsp balsamic vinegar

Preparations

- STEP 1

Mix all the ingredients for the salad and set aside. Heat 1 tsp oil in a large non-stick pan and fry the garlic briefly. Stir in the spinach to wilt, then mix in the tomato purée, tuna and cottage cheese. Set aside.

• STEP 2

Beat the eggs with the flour and 2 tbsp water. Heat the remaining oil in a medium non-stick pan, add half the batter and swirl round the pan to coat the base. Cook briefly until set, then flip over with a palate knife to cook the other side for 1 min. Repeat with the remaining batter. Put the pancakes on serving plates, spoon the filling down one side, roll up and serve with the salad.

Cheshire cheese, spinach & watercress salad

Ingredients

- 4 tbsp olive oil

- 2 tsp wholegrain mustard

- 1large red onion, very finely sliced

- 4 oranges

- 175g baby spinach

- 85g bag of watercress

- 225g Cheshire cheese or Wensleydale cheese, cut into chunks

- 100g blanched almond, split in half

- crusty bread, to serve

<u>**Preparations**</u>

- STEP 1

Mix the oil and mustard in a large salad bowl with salt and black pepper to taste. Add the red onion, stir well and allow to marinate while you prepare the oranges. The onion will soften and release a rosy colour into the dressing.

- STEP 2

Peel the oranges using a serrated knife and removing all the pith. Do this over the salad bowl so you catch all the juice. Segment the oranges with the knife to remove all the membrane, adding the segments to the bowl with the juice as you go.

• STEP 3

Toss the spinach, watercress and chunks of cheese with the oranges and dressing until they're all evenly coated.

• STEP 4

Now dry fry the almonds in a heavy frying pan, stirring them frequently until they begin to toast lightly. Tip the nuts on to the salad while they're still hot and serve immediately, with crusty bread to mop up the juices.

Niçoise chicken salad

<u>Ingredients</u>

For the dressing

- 2 tbsp rapeseed oil

- juice 1 lemon

- 1 tsp balsamic vinegar

- 1 garlic clove, grated

- ⅓ small pack basil, leaves chopped

- 3 pitted black Kalamata olive, rinsed and chopped

For the salad

- 2 skinless chicken breasts

- 1 tsp rapeseed oil

- 250g new potatoes, thickly sliced

- 200g fine green beans

- ½ red onion, very finely chopped

- 14 cherry tomatoes, halved

- 6 romaine lettuces leaves, torn into bite-sized pieces

- 6 pitted black Kalamata olive, rinsed and halved

<u>Preparations</u>

- STEP 1

Mix the dressing **<u>Ingredients</u>** together in a small bowl with 1 tbsp water. Add 1 tbsp of the dressing to the chicken breasts and toss well to coat. Heat the oil in a small non-stick frying pan with a lid and cook the chicken for about 12 mins, covered, turning over halfway until cooked all the way through.

• STEP 2

Meanwhile, boil the potatoes for 7 mins, add the beans and boil for 5 mins more or until both are just tender, then drain.

• STEP 3

Put the chicken on a plate to rest while you toss the beans, potatoes and remaining salad **Ingredients** together in a large bowl with half the dressing. Slice the chicken, arrange on the salad, then add any juices to the remaining dressing and spoon on top.

Sticky chicken & chorizo skewers

<u>Ingredients</u>

For the skewers

• 100ml olive oil

• 75ml sherry vinegar

• ½ small bunch thyme, leaves picked

• 1½ tbsp smoked paprika

• 4 garlic cloves, crushed

• 3 tbsp honey

• 4-5 chicken breasts (about 650g), cut into bite-sized chunks

- 200g chorizo ring, sliced into thick coins

- 250g padron pepper, or 3 green peppers cut into pieces

- charred lemon halves or wedges, to serve

For the olive oil flatbreads

- 1.2kg strong white bread flour, plus extra for dusting

- 200ml olive oil, plus extra for proving

- 1 tbsp fine salt

- 2 x 7g sachets fast-action dried yeast

Preparations

- STEP 1

Whisk the olive oil, vinegar, thyme, paprika, garlic and 2 tbsp honey with plenty of black pepper. Pour ¾ of the marinade over the chicken and chorizo, reserving the rest to glaze the skewers later. Marinate for at least 2 hrs or overnight. Whisk the leftover 1 tbsp honey into the reserved marinade.

• STEP 2

To make the flatbreads, mix the flour, olive oil, salt and yeast in a large bowl. Add 700ml water and knead to a rough dough. Tip onto a floured work surface and knead for 10 mins until smooth and elastic. Transfer to an oiled bowl and cover. Leave to double in size, about 1 hr.

• STEP 3

Knock the dough back and divide into 16 small balls about 140g each. Roll each out on a floured work surface until a few millimetres thick and about 20cm wide. Heat a dry frying pan on a medium high heat and cook the dough for 3-4 mins until golden underneath and large bubbles start forming. Flip and cook for 1-2 mins more until lightly golden. You can keep the flatbreads warm in a low oven or on the barbecue, wrapped in foil.

• STEP 4

Thread the chicken, chorizo and peppers onto eight large or 16 small metal skewers. Season with salt. Light a barbecue, let the flames die down and the coals turn ashy white, or heat the grill to medium high. Grill the skewers for 8-10 mins, turning every few mins until the chicken is cooked through. Use the remaining marinade to glaze the meat when turning.

• STEP 5

With a fork, slide the meat and peppers off the skewers on to the flatbreads. Serve sides separately for guests to assemble their own kebabs.

Chicken & avocado salad with blueberry balsamic dressing

Ingredients

• 1 garlic clove

• 85g blueberries

• 1 tbsp extra virgin rapeseed oil

- 2 tsp balsamic vinegar

- 125g fresh or frozen baby broad beans

- 1 large cooked beetroot, finely chopped

- 1 avocado, stoned, peeled and sliced

- 85g bag mixed baby leaf salad

- 175g cooked chicken

Preparations

- STEP 1

Finely chop the garlic. Mash half the blueberries with the oil, vinegar and some black pepper in a large salad bowl.

- STEP 2

Boil the broad beans for 5 mins until just tender. Drain, leaving them unskinned.

• STEP 3

Stir the garlic into the dressing, then pile in the warm beans and remaining blueberries with the beetroot, avocado, salad and chicken. Toss to mix, but don't go overboard or the juice from the beetroot will turn everything pink. Pile onto plates or into shallow bowls to serve.

Bean & quinoa salad with orange

Ingredients

• 120g quinoa

• 320g celery, strings removed if tough, sliced

- 320g frozen soya beans

- 2 tbsp extra virgin olive oil

- 3 tbsp apple cider vinegar

- 8 spring onions, trimmed and thinly sliced

- 30g flat-leaf parsley, chopped

- 4 tbsp chopped mint (optional)

- 4 small oranges, peeled and segmented

- 120g feta, crumbled

Preparations

- STEP 1

Tip the quinoa and celery into a pan and cover with plenty of water. Bring to the boil, then reduce the heat and simmer for 10 mins. Add the soya beans, bring back to the boil and cook for 7 mins more. Drain well, tip into a bowl and set aside.

• STEP 2

Add the oil, vinegar and spring onions, and leave to cool slightly before stirring in the parsley and mint. Serve two portions topped with half the segmented oranges and half the feta crumbled over. Chill the remaining salad for another day, then segment the remaining oranges and crumble over the feta just before serving. Will keep chilled in an airtight container for up to three days.

Wild salmon with corn & pepper salsa salad

<u>Ingredients</u>

For the spicy salmon

- 1 garlic clove

- ½ tsp mild chilli powder

- ½ tsp ground coriander

- ¼ tsp ground cumin

- 1 lime, grated zest and juice, plus wedges to serve (optional)

- 2 tsp rapeseed oil

- 2 wild salmon fillets

For the salsa salad

- 1 corn on the cob, husk removed if attached

- 1 red onion, finely chopped

- 1 avocado, stoned, peeled and finely chopped

- 1 red pepper, deseeded and finely chopped

- 1 red chilli, halved, deseeded and chopped

- ½ pack coriander, finely chopped

Preparations

- STEP 1

Finely grate the garlic into a bowl for the spice rub.
Boil the corn for the salsa salad for 6-8 mins until

tender, then drain and cut off the kernels with a sharp knife.

• STEP 2

Stir the spices, 1 tbsp lime juice and the oil into the garlic to make a spice rub, then use to coat the salmon.

• STEP 3

Mix the remaining lime zest and juice into the corn and stir in all the remaining **Ingredients** . Heat a frying pan and cook the salmon for 2 mins each side so that it is still a little pink in the centre. Serve with the salsa salad with extra lime wedges, if you like, for squeezing over.

Hummus & avocado sandwich topper

Ingredients

- 2 big spoonfuls hummus

- ½ small avocado, diced

- squeeze of lemon

- some chopped red onion

- coriander leaves

- some halved cherry tomatoes

- slice wholegrain seeded bread or rye, or wholegrain pitta, to serve

Preparations

• STEP 1

Top bread or fill pitta with hummus, then add avocado with lemon, red onion, coriander and cherry tomatoes.

Easy quinoa stir-fry

<u>Ingredients</u>

• 100g dried quinoa

• 1 tbsp sesame oil

• 1 small red onion, thinly sliced

• 1 garlic clove, grated

• thumb-sized piece ginger, grated

- ½ tsp ground coriander

- 1 tbsp wheat-free tamari

- 1 red pepper, cut in 1cm/ 1/2 slices

- 1 large courgette (about 250g/9oz), sliced

- 100g green beans, tailed and cut in half

- 2 tbsp sesame seeds

- small pack coriander, roughly chopped

For the dressing

- zest and juice 2 limes

- pinch of pink Himalayan salt

- 2 tbsp sesame oil

- ½ garlic clove, crushed

- ½ tsp brown rice vinegar

- 1 tsp wheat-free tamari

Preparations

- STEP 1

Cook the quinoa following pack instructions and leave to cool.

- STEP 2

In a large frying pan or wok, pour in the sesame oil, onion, garlic, ginger, ground coriander and tamari and fry on a medium-high heat for 2 mins until the moisture starts to evaporate, then add 3 tbsp water. Leave to fry for 1 min more, add the pepper and fry for another 2 mins.

• STEP 3

Add 4 tbsp water then after 2 mins, add the green beans and 125ml water.

• STEP 4

After another 2 mins, add the courgette, 125ml water and leave to cook for 3 mins, then take off the heat.

• STEP 5

Make the dressing by putting all the **Ingredients** in a jug and whisking until smooth. Mix the quinoa into the veg, add the dressing and mix together

with the sesame seeds. Stir through the coriander
to serve.

DINNER

Spinach crespolini

Ingredients

- 50g spelt wholemeal flour

- 1 egg

- 100ml milk

- ½ tsp rapeseed oil

- 250g baby spinach

- generous grating of nutmeg

- 1 large garlic clove, finely grated

• 80g ricotta

• 2 tbsp vegetarian Italian-style hard cheese, finely
grated

For the sauce

• 400g can chopped tomatoes

• 10g basil

• ½ tsp vegetable bouillon powder

• 1 garlic clove, crushed

For the salad

• 2 tsp balsamic vinegar

• 1 small red onion (about 80g), finely chopped

- 80g diced celery

- 3 handfuls of rocket

- 160g cherry tomatoes

<u>Preparations</u>

- STEP 1

Whisk the flour and egg together, then gradually whisk in the milk to create a smooth pancake-style batter. Pour into a jug.

- STEP 2

Heat the oil in a 19cm non-stick pan over a medium heat, tip in a quarter of the batter, and swirl to cover the base. Cook briefly until just set, then flip over using a palette knife and cook the other side until just golden. Lift onto a plate, then repeat with the remaining batter to make four pancakes in total.

• STEP 3

Meanwhile, heat a second large non-stick pan over a medium heat and cook the spinach, nutmeg and garlic for about 5 mins, stirring with a wooden spoon until the spinach has completely wilted. Remove from the heat and cool slightly, then beat in the ricotta. Spoon a quarter of the spinach filling down the centre of each pancake, then roll up into a sausage and arrange snugly in an ovenproof dish. Heat the oven to 200C/180C fan/gas 6.

• STEP 4

To make the sauce, put the canned tomatoes, basil, bouillon and garlic in a bowl, and blitz using a hand blender until completely smooth (or do this in a jug blender). Pour the sauce over the pancakes and scatter over the cheese. Bake for 30 mins until browned and bubbling at the edges. For the salad, combine the vinegar, onion and celery. Just before serving, toss the onion mixture with the rocket and tomatoes, and serve with the filled pancakes.

Spinach & barley risotto

Ingredients

• 2 tsp rapeseed oil

• 1 large leek (315g), thinly sliced

• 2 garlic cloves, chopped

• 2 x 400g can barley, undrained

• 1 tbsp vegetable bouillon powder

• 1 tsp finely chopped sage

• 1 tbsp thyme leaves

• 160g cherry tomatoes, halved

• 160g spinach

• 50g finely grated vegetarian Italian-style hard cheese

Preparations

• STEP 1

Heat the oil in a non-stick pan and fry the leek and garlic for 5-10 mins, stirring frequently, until softened, adding a splash of water if it sticks.

- STEP 2

Tip in the cans of barley and their liquid, then stir in the bouillon powder, sage and thyme. Simmer, stirring frequently, for 4-5 mins. Add the tomatoes and spinach and cook for 2-3 mins more until the spinach is wilted, adding a splash more water if needed. Stir in most of the cheese, then serve with the remaining cheese scattered over.

Egg wraps with black beans & rocket

Ingredients

- 1 red pepper, deseeded and sliced

- 2 tsp rapeseed or olive oil

- 1 garlic clove, finely grated

- ½ tsp ground cumin

- 1 tsp ground coriander

- 1 tsp vegetable bouillon powder

- 400g can black beans

For the wraps

- 4 large eggs

- handful of chopped parsley or coriander

- 4 tbsp porridge oats

- 2 tomatoes, chopped

- 2 handfuls of rocket

Preparations

• STEP 1

Put the pepper in a large non-stick pan with 1 tsp of the oil. Cover and cook over a medium heat for 10 mins, stirring occasionally. Add the garlic and spices, then tip in the bouillon and beans, along with the water in the can, then cook for a few minutes, stirring until slightly reduced. Mash the beans a couple of times to thicken the mixture.

• STEP 2

For the wraps, beat 2 eggs in a bowl with half the parsley or coriander and half the oats. Heat half the remaining oil in a 21cm non-stick frying pan, and fry the egg mixture for 1 min 30 seconds until almost set, then turn over. Fry for another 30-60 seconds. Tip onto a plate, spoon half the filling down the centre and scatter over half the tomato and rocket, then roll up and serve. Repeat the process with the rest of the ingredients to make the other wrap.

Honey mustard grilled salmon with puy lentils

Ingredients

- 1 lemon, zested and juiced

- 2 tsp wholegrain mustard

- 1 tbsp clear honey

- 2 skinless salmon fillets

- 2 tsp rapeseed oil

- 5 spring onions, sliced

- 175g cooked beetroot (not in vinegar), diced

- 250g pack ready-to-eat puy lentils

- 10 basil leaves

- 2 big handfuls rocket

<u>Preparations</u>

- STEP 1

Turn the grill to high and line a baking tray with foil. Mix the lemon zest and juice, mustard and honey. Put the salmon on the tray, brush with a little of the dressing, then grill for 5-7 mins – there is no need to turn the salmon over until it flakes easily when tested with a knife.

- STEP 2

Meanwhile, heat the oil in a wok and cook the spring onions and beetroot. Tip in the lentils with 4 tbsp water, cover the pan and cook for 2 mins to heat through. Tip into a bowl and toss with the remaining dressing, the basil and rocket. Serve with the salmon.

Cod & prawn pie with saffron potatoes

<u>Ingredients</u>

- 1 tbsp olive oil

- 1 yellow and red pepper, both deseeded and finely chopped

- 2 large garlic cloves, chopped

- 2 bay leaves

- 1 tbsp smoked paprika

- 150ml vegetable stock, made with 2 tsp bouillon powder

- 500g carton passata

- 240g pack frozen raw, peeled, large wild red shrimp, defrosted

- 2 x 280g packs skinless cod loin, cut into large chunks

- 9 pitted green olives, quartered (we used Amfissa olives, as they have a firmer texture)

- 3 tbsp chopped flat-leaf parsley (optional)

- 320g broccoli florets or green beans

For the saffron potatoes

- 3 generous pinches of saffron threads (about ⅓ x 0.5g sachet)

- 1 ½ tbsp olive oil

- 2 large garlic cloves, finely grated

- 725g large potatoes (about 4), peeled and thinly sliced

Preparations

- STEP 1

Heat the oven to 200C/180C fan/ gas 6. Warm the olive oil in a large non-stick pan over a medium heat and fry the peppers, garlic and bay leaves for

10 mins, stirring often until the peppers have softened.

• STEP 2

Meanwhile, prepare the saffron potatoes. Put the saffron threads in a small heatproof bowl with 1 tbsp boiling water, the olive oil and garlic, and stir well until the liquid turns yellow. Set aside. Bring a large pan of water to the boil, and cook the sliced potatoes for 5 mins until tender but not collapsing. Drain well.

• STEP 3

When the peppers have softened, sprinkle over the paprika and stir briefly, then pour in the stock and passata and cook for 5 mins more. Remove from the heat and stir in the shrimp, cod, olives and parsley, if using. Tip the stew into a large, shallow pie dish (ours was 30 x 20cm, and about 6.5cm deep).

• STEP 4

Arrange the potato slices over the stew in an even layer – they don't have to be neat – then generously brush over the saffron mixture.

• STEP 5

Bake the pie for 30-35 mins until bubbling at the edges and the fish is cooked through. When it's almost finished cooking, boil or steam the broccoli or green beans to serve alongside the pie.

South American-style quinoa with fried eggs

<u>Ingredients</u>

• 75g quinoa

• 400g can black beans, drained

• ½ tsp ground cumin

• ½ tsp ground coriander

• 1 lime, zested and juiced, plus extra wedges to serve

• 1 tsp cider vinegar

• 160g cherry tomatoes, halved

• 1 small avocado, stoned, peeled and roughly chopped

• 2 tbsp finely chopped coriander

- 3 spring onions or ½ small red onion, finely chopped

- rapeseed oil, for frying

- 2 medium eggs

<u>Preparations</u>

- STEP 1

Put the quinoa in a small pan with 250ml water and bring to the boil. Reduce the heat to low, cover and gently simmer for 15-20 mins, stirring occasionally until most of the water has been absorbed and the grains have doubled in size (if there's any water left in the pan, drain well).

- STEP 2

Tip into a bowl and stir through the beans, spices, lime zest and juice and vinegar. Stir well, then add the tomatoes, avocado, coriander and onion, and spoon onto plates.

• STEP 3

Heat a drop of oil in a non-stick frying pan and fry the eggs until the whites are set with a crispy edge and the yolk is runny. Serve the quinoa topped with the eggs.

Healthy chicken stir-fry

Ingredients

• 65g brown basmati rice

• 2 tsp rapeseed oil

- 15g ginger, peeled and cut into thin matchsticks

- 2 small red onions (160g), cut into wedges

- 160g broccoli, broken into florets, stem finely chopped

- 2 carrots (160g), halved lengthways, then cut into diagonal slices

- 1 red chilli, finely chopped (optional)

- 200g chicken breast, cut into thin strips

- ½ tsp ground cumin

- 1 tbsp crunchy peanut butter

- 1 tbsp wheat-free tamari

- 1 tbsp brown rice vinegar

Preparations

• STEP 1

Cook the rice following pack instructions, then drain. Heat the oil in a non-stick wok over a high heat and fry the ginger and red onions for 2 mins. Add the broccoli stem, carrots and chilli, if using, and cook for 1 min.

• STEP 2

Tip in the chicken and cumin, stir-fry briefly, then add the broccoli florets and 3 tbsp water. Cover and leave to steam for 3-4 mins, or until the broccoli florets are just tender and the chicken is cooked through.

• STEP 3

Meanwhile, mix the peanut butter with the tamari and vinegar. Stir the sauce into the veg and chicken, then serve over the cooked rice.

Pepper & mushroom socca pizza

<u>Ingredients</u>

• 1 tsp rapeseed oil

• 70g mushrooms, thinly sliced

• 1 pepper, halved, deseeded and thinly sliced

• 2 tbsp tomato purée

• 1 garlic clove, finely grated

• 2 tomatoes, chopped

- 2 tbsp chopped basil

- 30g grated mature cheddar

For the base

- 160g chickpea (gram) flour

- 1 tbsp rapeseed oil

<u>Preparations</u>

- STEP 1

Heat the oven to 200C/180C fan/gas 6. For the base, put the flour in a large bowl. Whisk in 250ml water to make a batter. Heat the oil in a large, non-stick frying pan. Pour in the batter and cook over a low heat for 4-5 mins until set. Loosen with a palate knife or spatula, turn and cook for 1-2 mins on the other side.

• STEP 2

Meanwhile, for the toppings, heat the oil in a pan over a medium heat and stir-fry the mushrooms and peppers until soft, about 4-5 mins. Mix the tomato purée and garlic in a bowl with 2 tbsp water, then stir in the chopped tomatoes.

• STEP 3

Turn the base out onto a baking tray lined with baking parchment. Spread over the tomato mixture. Scatter over the mushrooms, peppers, half the basil and the cheese. Bake for 5-10 mins until the cheese has melted. Scatter with the remaining basil to serve.

Spicy fish stew

<u>Ingredients</u>

• 1 tbsp olive oil

• 2 onions, thinly sliced

• 3 spring onions, chopped

• 3 garlic cloves, chopped

• 1 red chilli, seeded and thinly sliced

• few thyme sprigs

• 2 x 400g cans chopped tomatoes

• 400ml vegetable bouillon made with 2 tsp vegetable bouillon powder

• 2 green peppers, seeded and cut into pieces

• 160g brown basmati rice

• 400g can and 210g can red kidney beans, drained

• handful fresh coriander, chopped, plus a few sprigs extra

• handful flat-leaf parsley, chopped

• 550g pack frozen wild salmon, skinned and cut into large pieces

• 1 lime, zested

Preparations

• STEP 1

Heat the oil in a large non-stick pan and fry the onions for 8-10 mins until softened and golden. Add the spring onions, garlic, chilli and thyme. Cook, stirring, for 1 min. Pour in the tomatoes and bouillon, then stir in the peppers. Cover and leave to simmer for 15 mins.

• STEP 2

Meanwhile, cook the rice according to pack instructions. Stir in the beans with the coriander and parsley, then leave to cook gently for another 10 mins until the peppers are tender. Add the salmon and lime zest and cook for 4-5 mins until cooked through.

• STEP 3

Ladle into bowls and scatter with the coriander sprigs.

Salmon salad with sesame dressing

<u>**Ingredients**</u>

For the salad

- 250g new potatoes, sliced

- 160g French beans, trimmed

- 2 wild salmon fillets

- 80g salad leaves

- 4 small clementines, 3 sliced, 1 juiced

- handful of basil, chopped

- handful of coriander, chopped

For the dressing

- 2 tsp sesame oil

- 2 tsp tamari

- ½ lemon, juiced

- 1 red chilli, deseeded and chopped

- 2 tbsp finely chopped onion (¼ small onion)

Preparations

- STEP 1

Steam the potatoes and beans in a steamer basket set over a pan of boiling water for 8 mins. Arrange the salmon fillets on top and steam for a further 6-8 mins, or until the salmon flakes easily when tested with a fork.

- STEP 2

Meanwhile, mix the dressing **Ingredients** together along with the clementine juice. If eating straightaway, divide the salad leaves between two plates and top with the warm potatoes and beans and the clementine slices. Arrange the salmon fillets on top, scatter over the herbs and spoon over the dressing. If taking to work, prepare the potatoes, beans and salmon the night before, then pack into a rigid airtight container with the salad leaves kept separate. Put the salad elements together and dress just before eating to prevent the leaves from wilting.

Black bean tortilla with salsa

Ingredients

For the salsa

- 400g can chopped tomatoes

- 1 onion, finely chopped

- 1 red chilli, halved, deseeded and finely chopped

- 2 tsp smoked paprika

- 15g (1/2 pack) coriander, finely chopped

- 6 Kalamata olives, thinly sliced

- ½ lemon or lime, juiced

For the omelette

- 2 x 400g can black beans, drained

- 3 garlic cloves, finely grated

- 2 tsp ground cumin

- 2 tsp ground coriander

- 6 large eggs

- 1 tbsp rapeseed oil

- 4 generous handfuls of rocket

<u>Preparations</u>

- STEP 1

Tip the tomatoes into a pan and stir in the onion, ½ the chilli and the smoked paprika. Cook over a low heat for 10 mins. Tip ¾ into a bowl, then stir in 2 tbsp of the coriander and the olives and lemon juice.

- STEP 2

Meanwhile, heat the grill. Tip the beans into a bowl and stir in the remaining chilli, the garlic, cumin and coriander. Beat in the eggs, then add the reserved ¼ of the salsa and the remaining fresh coriander with a little salt to taste. Blitz a little using a hand blender or mash some of the beans with a potato masher.

• STEP 3

Heat a 24cm non-stick pan with the oil. Pour in the bean mixture and leave to cook gently for 5-7 mins until the base is set, then grill for 5 mins. Tip out and cut into 4 wedges.

Spiced chicken with rice & crisp red onions

<u>Ingredients</u>

• 2 boneless skinless chicken breasts, about 140g/5oz each

• 1 tbsp sunflower oil

• 2 tsp curry powder

• 1 large red onion, thinly sliced

• 100g basmati rice

• 1 cinnamon stick

• pinch saffron

• 1 tbsp raisins

• 85g frozen pea

• 1 tbsp chopped mint and coriander

• 4 rounded tbsp low-fat natural yogurt

Preparations

• STEP 1

Heat oven to 190C/fan 170C/gas 5. Brush the chicken with 1 tsp oil, then sprinkle with curry powder. Toss the onion in the remaining oil. Put the chicken and onions in one layer in a roasting tin. Bake for 25 mins until the meat is cooked and the onions are crisp, stirring the onions halfway through the cooking time.

• STEP 2

Rinse the rice, then put in a pan with the cinnamon, saffron, salt to taste and 300ml water. Bring to the boil, stir once, add the raisins, cover. Gently cook for 10-12 mins until the rice is tender, adding the peas halfway through. Spoon the rice onto two plates, top with the chicken and scatter over the onions. Stir the herbs into the yogurt and season, if you like, before serving on the side.

One-pot vegan rice and beans

<u>Ingredients</u>

• 2 tbsp rapeseed oil

• 2 onions (320g), finely chopped

• 1 orange pepper, halved, deseeded and cut into 4-5 chunky pieces

• 1 red pepper, halved, deseeded and cut into 4-5 chunky pieces

• 3 large garlic cloves, sliced

* 300g easy-cook brown rice

* 1 tbsp thyme leaves

* 2 tbsp smoked paprika

* 650ml hot vegetable stock, made with 2 tsp vegetable bouillon powder

* 10 pitted green olives

* 400g can red kidney beans, drained

* ½ lemon, cut into wedges

Preparations

* STEP 1

Heat the oil in a large saucepan over a medium heat and fry the onions for 5 mins, stirring frequently until softened. Add the peppers and garlic and cook for 5 mins more, stirring every now and then.

• STEP 2

Tip in the rice, thyme and paprika, then pour in the stock and stir in the olives. Cover and leave to cook over a low heat for 15 mins. Stir in the kidney beans, then cover and cook for 20-30 mins more until the rice is tender. Top with the lemon wedges, then cover and leave for 5 mins. Spoon two portions into bowls and serve. Cool and chill the remainder to eat another day. Will keep chilled for one day. To serve, reheat in a pan or in the microwave until piping hot (remove the lemon wedges before heating).

Hake & seafood cataplana

Ingredients

- 2 tbsp cold-pressed rapeseed oil

- 1 onion, halved and thinly sliced

- 250g salad potatoes, cut into chunks

- 1 large red pepper, deseeded and chopped

- 1 courgette (200g), thickly sliced

- 2 tomatoes, chopped (150g)

- 2 large garlic cloves, finely grated

- 1 tbsp cider vinegar (optional)

- 2 tsp vegetable bouillon powder

• 2 skinless hake fillets (pack size 240g)

• 150g pack ready-cooked mussels (not in shells)

• 60g peeled prawns

• large handful of parsley, chopped

Preparations

• STEP 1

Heat the oil in a wide non-stick pan with a tight-fitting lid. Fry the onions and potatoes for about 5 mins, or until starting to soften. Add the peppers, courgettes, tomatoes and garlic, then stir in the vinegar, if using, the bouillon and 200ml water. Bring to a simmer, cover and cook for 25 mins, or until the peppers and courgettes are very tender (if your pan doesn't have a tight-fitting lid, wet a sheet of baking parchment and place over the stew before covering – this helps keep in the juices).

• STEP 2

Add the hake fillets, mussels and prawns, then cover and cook for 5 mins more, or until the fish flakes easily when tested with a fork. Scatter over the parsley and serve.

SNACKS RECIPES FOR NUTRISYSTEM DIET

Double ginger cookies

Ingredients

- 350g plain flour

- 1 tbsp ground ginger

- 1 tsp bicarbonate of soda

- 175g light muscovado sugar

- 100g butter, chopped

- 8 pieces of stem ginger, chopped (not too finely), plus thin slices, to decorate (optional)

- 1 large egg

- 4 tbsp golden syrup

- 200g bar dark chocolate, chopped

<u>Preparations</u>

- STEP 1

Mix the flour, ground ginger, bicarbonate of soda, 1/2 tsp salt and sugar in a bowl, then rub in the butter to make crumbs. Stir in the chopped stem ginger.

- STEP 2

Beat together the egg and syrup, pour into the dry **<u>Ingredients</u>** and stir, then knead with your hands to make a dough. Cut the dough in half and shape each piece into a thick sausage about 6cm across, making sure that the ends are straight. Wrap in cling film and chill for 20 mins. You can now freeze all or part of the dough for 2 months.

• STEP 3

Heat oven to 180C/160C fan/gas 4 and line 2 baking sheets with baking parchment. Thickly slice each sausage into 12 and put the slices on the baking sheets, spacing them well apart and reshaping any, if necessary, to make rounds. Bake for 12 mins, then leave to cool for a few mins to harden before transferring to a wire rack to cool completely.

• STEP 4

Melt the chocolate in a bowl over a pan of gently simmering water, making sure that the water isn't touching the bottom of the bowl. Dip half of each cookie into the chocolate – you may need to spoon it over when you get to the final few. Decorate with a slice of ginger, if you like, and leave to set. Will keep for 1 week in an airtight container.

Homemade vegan bagels

<u>Ingredients</u>

- 7g sachet dried yeast

- 4 tbsp sugar

- 2 tsp salt

- 450g bread flour

- poppy, fennel and/or sesame seeds to sprinkle on top (optional)

Preparations

- STEP 1

Tip the yeast and 1 tbsp sugar into a large bowl, and pour over 100ml warm water. Leave for 10 mins until the mixture becomes frothy.

- STEP 2

Pour 200ml warm water into the bowl, then stir in the salt and half the flour. Keep adding the remaining flour (you may not have to use it all) and mixing with your hands until you have a soft but not sticky dough. Then knead for 10 mins until the dough feels smooth and elastic. Shape into a ball and put in a clean, lightly oiled bowl. Cover loosely and leave in a warm place until doubled in size, about 1hr.

• STEP 3

Heat the oven to 220C/200C fan/gas 7. On a lightly floured surface, divide the dough into 10 pieces, each about 85g. Shape each piece into a flattish ball, then take a wooden spoon and use the handle to make a hole in the middle of each ball. Slip the spoon into the hole, then twirl the bagel around the spoon to make a hole about 3cm wide. Cover the bagel loosely while you shape the remaining dough.

• STEP 4

Meanwhile, bring a large pan of water to the boil and tip in the remaining sugar. Slip the bagels into the boiling water – no more than four at a time. Cook for 1-2 mins, turning over in the water until the bagels have puffed slightly and a skin has formed. Remove with a slotted spoon and drain away any excess water. Sprinkle over your choice of topping and place on a baking tray lined with parchment. Bake in the oven for 25 mins until browned and crisp – the bases should sound hollow when tapped. Leave to cool on a wire rack, then serve with your favourite filling.

Flat apple & vanilla tart

<u>Ingredients</u>

- 375g pack puff pastry, preferably all-butter

- 5 large eating apples - Cox's, russets or Elstar

- juice of 1 lemon

- 25g butter, cut into small pieces

- 3 tsp vanilla sugar or 1 tsp vanilla extract

• 1 tbsp caster sugar

• 3 rounded tbsp apricot conserve

Preparations

• STEP 1

Heat oven to 220C/fan 200C/gas 7. Roll out the pastry and trim to a round about 35cm across. Transfer to a baking sheet lined with parchment paper.

• STEP 2

Peel, core and thinly slice the apples and toss in the lemon juice. Spread over the pastry to within 2cm of the edges. Curl up the edges slightly to stop the juices running off.

- STEP 3

Dot the top with the butter and sprinkle with vanilla and caster sugar. Bake for 15-20 mins until the apples are tender and the pastry crisp.

- STEP 4

Warm the conserve and brush over the apples and pastry edge. Serve hot with vanilla ice cream or crème fraîche.

Puff pastry pizzas

Ingredients

- 320g sheet ready-rolled light puff pastry

- 6 tbsp tomato purée

* 1 tbsp tomato ketchup

* 1 tsp dried oregano

* 75g mozzarella or cheddar

For the topping

* sweetcorn, olives, peppers, red onion, cherry tomatoes, spinach, basil

Preparations

* STEP 1

Heat the oven to 200C/180C fan/gas 6, or if using an air-fryer, heat it to 180C for 4 mins. Unroll the pastry, cut into six squares and arrange over two baking trays lined with baking parchment. Use a cutlery knife to score a 1cm border around the edge of each pastry square. Bake in the oven for 15 mins, until puffed up but not cooked through. Or, if using an air-fryer, bake the batch for 8 mins. You might need to do this in two batches.

• STEP 2

While the pastry cooks, make the sauce and prepare your toppings. Mix the tomato purée, tomato ketchup, oregano and 1 tbsp water. Grate the cheese and chop any veg or herbs you want to put on top into small pieces. Set aside.

• STEP 3

Remove the pastry from the oven or air-fryer and squash down the middles with the back of a spoon. Divide the sauce between the pastry squares and spread it out to the puffed-up edges. Sprinkle with the cheese, then add your toppings. Bake for another 5-8 mins in the oven or 5 mins in the air-fryer and serve.

Glamorous fairy cakes

<u>Ingredients</u>

For the cakes

- 140g butter, very well softened

- 140g golden caster sugar

- 3 medium eggs

- 100g self-raising flour

- 25g custard powder or cornflour

For decorating

- 600g icing sugar, sifted

- 6 tbsp water, or half water and half lemon juice, strained

- edible green and pink food colourings

- crystallised violets

- crystallised roses or rose petals

- edible wafer flowers

Preparations

- STEP 1

Heat the oven to 190C/fan 170C/gas 5. Arrange paper cases in bun tins. Put all the cake **Ingredients** in a large bowl and beat for about 2 mins until smooth. Divide the mixture between the cases so they are half filled and bake for 12-15 mins, until risen and golden. Cool on a wire rack.

• STEP 2

Mix the icing sugar and water until smooth and use a third on eight of the cakes. Divide the rest in half, and colour one half pale green and the other half pale pink. Decorate the white ones with crystallised violets, the pink ones with the roses and the green ones with the wafer flowers. Leave to set. Will keep for up to 2-3 days stored in an airtight container in a cool place.

Easy plum jam

Ingredients

• 2kg plums, stoned and roughly chopped

- 2kg white granulated sugar

- 2 tsp ground cinnamon

- 1 tbsp lemon juice

- 3 cinnamon sticks (optional)

- knob of butter

<u>Preparations</u>

- STEP 1

Sterilise the jars and any other equipment before you start (see tip). Put a couple of saucers in the freezer, as you'll need these for testing whether the jam is ready later (or use a sugar thermometer). Put the plums in a preserving pan and add 200ml water. Bring to a simmer, and cook for about 10 mins until the plums are tender but not falling apart. Add the sugar, ground cinnamon and lemon juice, then let the sugar dissolve slowly, without boiling. This will take about 10 mins.

• STEP 2

Increase the heat and bring the jam to a full rolling boil. After about 5 mins, spoon a little jam onto a cold saucer. Wait a few seconds, then push the jam with your fingertip. If it wrinkles, the jam is ready. If not, cook for a few mins more and test again, with another cold saucer. If you have a sugar thermometer, it will read 105C when ready.

• STEP 3

Take the jam off the heat and add the cinnamon sticks (if using) and the knob of butter. The cinnamon will look pretty in the jars and the butter will disperse any scum. Let the jam cool for 15 mins, which will prevent the lumps of fruit sinking to the bottom of the jars. Ladle into hot jars, seal and leave to cool. Will keep for 1 year in a cool, dark place. Chill once opened.

Freezer biscuits

Ingredients

- 200g pack butter, softened

- 200g soft brown sugar

- 2 eggs

- 1 tsp vanilla extract

- 200g self-raising flour

- 140g oats

Your choice of flavours

- 50g chopped nuts such as pecan, hazelnuts or almonds

- 50g desiccated coconut

- 50g raisin, or mixed fruit

<u>Preparations</u>

- STEP 1

When the butter is really soft, tip it into a bowl along with the sugar. Using an electric hand whisk or exercising some arm muscle, beat together until the sugar is mixed through. Beat in the eggs, one at a time, followed by the vanilla extract and a pinch of salt, if you like. Stir in the flour and oats. The mixture will be quite stiff at this point. Now decide what else you would like to add – any or all of the flavours are delicious – and stir through.

• STEP 2

Tear off an A4-size sheet of greaseproof paper. Pile up half the mixture in the middle of the sheet, then use a spoon to thickly spread the mixture along the centre of the paper. Pull over one edge of paper and roll up until you get a tight cylinder. If you have problems getting it smooth, then roll as you would a rolling pin along a kitchen surface. You'll need it to be about the width of a teacup. When it is tightly wrapped, twist up the ends and then place in the freezer. Can be frozen for up to 3 months.

• STEP 3

To cook, heat oven to 180C/fan 160C/gas 4 and unwrap the frozen biscuit mix. Using a sharp knife, cut off a disk about ½cm wide. If you have difficulty slicing through, dip the knife into a cup of hot water. Cut off as many biscuits as you need, then pop the mix back into the freezer for another time. Place on a baking sheet, spacing them widely apart as the mixture will spread when cooking, then cook for 15 mins until the tops are golden brown. Leave to cool for at least 5 mins before eating.

Instant berry banana slush

<u>Ingredients</u>

• 2 ripe bananas

• 200g frozen berry mix (blackberries, raspberries and currants)

Preparations

• STEP 1

Slice the bananas into a bowl and add the frozen berry mix. Blitz with a stick blender to make a slushy ice and serve straight away in two glasses with spoons.

Ricotta and basil pizza

Ingredients

• 1 onion, finely chopped

• 2 yellow peppers, roughly chopped

- 1 tsp olive oil

- 2 x 400g/14oz cans chopped tomatoes

- 500g bag mixed grain or granary bread mix

- plain flour, for dusting

- 10 cherry tomatoes, halved or whole

- 250g tub ricotta

- a few basil leaves, to serve

Preparations

- STEP 1

Heat oven to 220C/fan 200C/gas 6. Soften the onion and peppers in the oil in a large pan for a few mins. Pour in the tomatoes, season, then simmer for 10 mins.

• STEP 2

Meanwhile, make up the bread mix according to pack instructions, then bring the dough together and knead a couple of times. Flour a large baking sheet and roll out the dough into a rectangle roughly 25 x 35cm. Bake for 5 mins on a shelf at the top of the oven until firm.

• STEP 3

Remove from the oven, spread with the sauce, add the cherry tomatoes, then dollop over spoonfuls of the ricotta. Bake for 10 mins more until the base is golden and crisp. Scatter with basil and serve straight away with a green salad.

Mozzarella, pepper & aubergine calzone

Ingredients

- 400g strong wholewheat bread flour, plus extra for dusting

- ⅛ tsp salt (optional)

- 7g sachet fast-action dried yeast

- 2 tsp rapeseed oil, plus extra for the baking sheet

For the filling

- 2 tsp rapeseed oil

- 1 red and 1 yellow pepper, deseeded and cut into small chunks

- 1 large aubergine, halved lengthways and thinly sliced

- 2 large garlic cloves, finely chopped

- 1 tbsp tomato purée

- 1 tbsp balsamic vinegar

- small bunch basil, roughly torn

- 8 pitted Kalamata olives, halved

- 125g ball mozzarella (drained weight), quartered

- milk or beaten egg, for brushing

Preparations

- STEP 1

Put the flour, salt (if using), yeast, oil and 300ml lukewarm water in a bowl and mix until soft. Knead into a ball (try not to add any extra flour) – it will be sticky but the flour will absorb some moisture. Return to the bowl, cover and leave somewhere warm.

• STEP 2

Meanwhile, make the filling. Heat the oil in a large non-stick pan, then stir-fry the peppers for about 1 min until they start to soften. Add the aubergine and garlic and continue to cook over a medium heat for 8-10 mins, gently pressing the veg with a wooden spoon until it breaks down a little. If it doesn't, fry, covered, for a few extra mins.

• STEP 3

Stir in the tomato purée, vinegar and 2 tbsp water. When the veg is soft, remove the pan from the heat and stir through the basil.

• STEP 4

Heat the oven to 220C/200C fan/gas 7. Quarter the risen dough and roll each piece out to a 20cm circle on a lightly floured surface. Spoon a quarter of the filling over one side, scatter over a quarter of the olives, top with a quarter of the cheese, and brush the edges with the milk or beaten egg. Fold the dough over the filling and pinch the edges together at the side, a bit like making a Cornish pasty. Lift onto a lightly oiled baking sheet and brush with more milk or beaten egg. Repeat with the remaining dough and filling to make four calzones, then bake for 15-20 mins until golden.

Leave to cool slightly and serve at room temperature.

Spiced mackerel on toast with beetroot salsa

<u>Ingredients</u>

* 250g pack beetroot (not in vinegar), diced

* 1 eating apple, cut into wedges then thinly sliced

* 1 small red onion, finely sliced

* juice ½ lemon

* 1 tbsp olive oil, plus extra for drizzling

* 1 tsp cumin seed

* small bunch coriander, leaves roughly chopped

For the fish

- 4 mackerel fillets, halved widthways

- 1 tsp curry powder

- 4 slices sourdough bread or ciabatta

Preparations

- STEP 1

Mix the beetroot, apple, onion, lemon juice, oil, cumin and coriander together, season well, then set aside while you cook the mackerel. Heat the grill to high. Put the fish onto a sheet of foil on the grill rack, sprinkle over the curry powder, drizzle with oil, then season and rub well into the fish.

- STEP 2

Grill for 4-5 mins until the skin is crisp and the fillets are cooked through; you won't need to turn the fish over. Toast the bread in a toaster or alongside the fish under the grill, then drizzle with a little olive oil. Top with the salsa and mackerel, then pour over any pan juices and eat straight away.

Korean fried chicken burgers

Ingredients

For the chicken

• 4 skinless boneless chicken thighs fillets

• large piece of ginger, finely grated

• 100g cornflour

- vegetable oil, for frying

For the sauce

- 6 tbsp dark brown sugar

- 2 tbsp Korean chilli paste (gochujang) – see tip

- 2 tbsp soy sauce

- 2 large garlic cloves, crushed

- small piece ginger, grated

- 2 tsp sesame oil

For the kimchi-style slaw

- ½ white cabbage, finely sliced

- 1 mooli, shredded into thin strips

- 4 spring onions, finely sliced

- small piece ginger, grated

- 1 tsp golden caster sugar

- 1 garlic clove, crushed

- 2 tbsp mayonnaise

- pinch of hot chilli powder

To serve

- 1 Little Gem lettuce, divided into leaves

- 4 brioche or sesame seed burger buns, split and lightly toasted

Preparations

- STEP 1

Make the slaw by combining all the ingredients together. Taste and add more chilli powder, if you like. Chill in the fridge.

- STEP 2

To make the sauce, put all the ingredients in a saucepan and simmer gently until syrupy. Take off the heat and set aside.

- STEP 3

Cut away any fatty excess from the chicken thighs, then season with salt, pepper and the grated ginger. Toss the chicken with the cornflour until completely coated.

- STEP 4

Heat about 2cm of vegetable oil in a large frying pan. Fry the chicken thighs for 4-5 mins each side until crisp. Remove from the oil onto kitchen paper and leave to cool slightly for 2 mins. Then re-fry in the hot oil until ultra-crisp and you can hear it crackle. Remove to kitchen paper to drain.

• STEP 5

Reheat the sauce. Build your burgers by placing some lettuce and kimchi slaw on the base of a bun, top with the crispy chicken and drizzle over the sticky sauce.

Vegetarian club

Ingredients

• 3 slices granary bread

- 1 large handful watercress

- 1 carrot, peeled and coarsely grated

- small squeeze lemon juice

- 1 tbsp olive oil

- 2 dessertspoons reduced-fat hummus

- 2 tomatoes, thickly sliced

Preparations

- STEP 1

Toast the bread. Meanwhile, mix the watercress, carrot, lemon juice and olive oil together. In a small bowl spread the hummus over each slice of toast. Top 1 slice with the watercress and carrot salad, sandwich with another slice of toast and top with the tomato. Lay the final slice of bread, hummus side down, then press down and eat as is or cut the sandwich into quarters.

Avocado & strawberry ices

Ingredients

• 200g ripe strawberries, hulled and chopped

• 1 avocado, stoned, peeled and roughly chopped

• 2 tsp balsamic vinegar

• ½ tsp vanilla extract

• 1-2 tsp maple syrup (optional)

Preparations

- STEP 1

Put the strawberries (save four pieces for the top), avocado, vinegar and vanilla in a bowl and blitz using a hand blender (or in a food processor) until as smooth as you can get it. Have a taste and only add the maple syrup if the strawberries are not sweet enough.

- STEP 2

Pour into containers, add a strawberry to each, cover with cling film and freeze. Allow the pots to soften for 5-10 mins before eating.

PART V

LIFESTYLE INTEGRATION AND LONG-TERM SUCCESS

Nutrisystem encourages people on the program to stay fit and exercise according to government recommendations, which is 150 minutes of moderate-intense activity per week. They encourage you to do 30 minutes of exercise five days per week. For people short on time, you can break up the 30 minutes into smaller 15- or 10-minute bouts. You're also encouraged to do two strength-training sessions per week.

Testimonials and Success Stories from Nutrisystem Users

Nutrisystem is a weight loss company that was founded in 1976 and has an A+ Better Business Bureau rating.

The company was involved in several lawsuits in the 1990s over concerns that the program's rapid weight loss regimen was potentially causing gallbladder disease in teens. The investigations have since been closed, and no new allegations have been made publicly.

Reviews of Nutrisystem are mixed. Satisfied customers report that they appreciate the convenience Nutrisystem offers and share that they were able to lose weight while following the diet.

However, several reviewers note that while they initially lost weight, they gained most of it back when the service became too expensive to continue using.

In addition to the cost, the most common complaints are about the food. Specifically, several reviewers mention that the meals are bland and too small to be satisfying. Some customers also report issues with meals arriving partially opened or containing moldy food.

Finally, many reviewers express frustration with Nutrisystem's customer service department, especially when trying to cancel their membership.